I0479799

Messages from the Spirit World

Telepathic messages with spirit activity away and at home.

Vol 4

Extract from the original book,

'A Glimpse in a Transient Zone'

Jo Eaton.

Copyright.

All rights reserved. No part of this book may be reproduced by any mechanical, photographic, or electronic process, or in the form of a phonographic recording; nor may it be stored in a retrieval system, transmitted, or otherwise be copied for public or private use - other than for 'fair use' as brief quotations embodied in articles and reviews - without prior written permission of the publisher.

Disclaimer.

The author of this book does not dispense medical advice or prescribe the use of any technique as a form of treatment for physical or medical problems without the advice of a physician, either directly or indirectly. The intent of the author is only to offer information of a general nature to help you in your quest for emotional and spiritual well-being. In the event you use any of the information in this book for yourself, which Is your constitutional right, the author and the publisher assume no responsibility for your actions.

In order to protect identity, I have changed the names of some of the characters within many of the stories.

Contents

Chapter 1

Telepathic Messages from the Spirit World

I have read of poets who have had a 'mind blank', sitting in front of an empty piece of paper, then, suddenly, they start to write as though they are receiving a dictation. On completion, the poet is amazed at the outcome. Almost like there has been some Divine intervention. Personally, I have had this happen to me a few times. Once, I too wrote a poem, my first and last attempt. It was about the wildlife I encountered on a coastal walk in Pembrokeshire. The poem was lengthy and it seemed to write itself, without any effort from myself. I was shocked at the final outcome. Perhaps I ought to try writing more poems.

Throughout my journey, I know I am well taken care of, having guides and helpers giving me love and encouragement along the way. Some of the messages I have received have been from loved ones who have died. I remember being devastated following the death of my Mum, who had been terminally ill from cancer for eight years before she finally passed. We were extremely close emotionally and so her death left me bereft. I already had two young children at the time, when eighteen months later, I had a daughter. Walking to town one day, while pushing the pram, with tears streaming down my face, because I was still grieving the loss of my Mum, I heard a clear voice, my Mum's voice saying, 'Enough is enough'. Instinctively, I recognised the familiar voice and knew my Mum wanted an end to the grieving. She was fine and I needed to concentrate on raising my family and to live a full life. Even now, after forty years since that event, I can remember exactly the place where I heard this message.

Although my brother had lived in Germany for forty-five years, we had always been emotionally close and in constant contact, as we were the only siblings, since our parents had passed many years earlier. I know my brother 'visited' me while he lay in a hospital bed in Germany, suffering from a brain tumour. I asked," Hey, what are you doing here?" My brother replied, "Oh, it's OK over here". (I believe he was referring to the dimension we move to after our death). To which I replied, 'You had better go back because it is not yet your time'.

It was three weeks later, when my brother passed over, although I was aware of his passing being two o'clock in the early hours and yet officially the time was seven hours later, the time taken for his vital organs to shut down. There are still times when I miss my big brother, but I am comforted in the knowledge that we will meet up again sometime in the distant future.

There are some wonderful ways us humans communicate with each other, not always commonly acknowledged. Sometimes, I am awakened by someone who wishes to communicate messages to either me or some other person, whereby I am just the messenger. Mostly, this is not a problem, because I often have disturbed sleep being a light sleeper and so the following morning, I will usually write up about the conversation and forward any requests to the relevant friends or family. However, if I am tired or not well, I politely ask them to go away because I need to rest and I will talk to them another time. Spirit seems to acknowledge this request because they always return at some time later.

Sometimes, during the night, I may receive messages and communications when I am not asleep, but in a relaxed state, when my surroundings are extremely quiet. One such time, I heard clear healing instructions, as when I am performing Reiki or giving some healing, but the message in my left ear was the voice of a modern, youngish male, one who was extremely confident. I asked, "Who are you?" "It is I, the physician", came the reply. I immediately thought that reply sounded such an ancient phraseology, rather than the modern language used of today. When I later asked my guide the name of the physician, I was told, 'All in good time'.

I receive messages during the night and day, being reminded to contact someone who may be in need, particularly if a family member may be in danger. I always know immediately.

I have had many psychic events and visitations to confirm to me that friends and family who are no longer in the physical dimension, are able to visit us with messages of greetings. I know each of my close family have visited me and only a few years ago, one of my ear-rings lifted out of my ear and dropped a metre away onto the carpet. I have seen bath towels raised then drop back onto the rail, candles disappear, tops of sealed glass jar turned upside down etc. My family are not alarmed by such happenings. In fact, they are used to them, realising it is just acknowledgement of our nearest and dearest who are still around us, just vibrating on another frequency. In fact, I once asked my brother on one of his psychic visits to me, how did he know I was thinking about him. He said when you are communicating telepathically with the other side, when you mention a name, then a small bell rings, telling them to make contact with the physical realm. I have never read about this method of contact; it is just the message conveyed to me by my brother. This continuous communication with the other dimension is of great comfort as it acts as confirmation, we do not die but just pass through another energy system.

I remember one time when I was writing up my thesis on the topic of the spiritual content of the artist Monet's paintings. My printer was busy churning out the pages and yet when it came to the script regarding my observations of Monet's content, then my printer shuddered to a halt. After constantly attempting to print, changing inks, my husband's intervention as to the mechanics of the printer, (something he was very familiar as part of his daily job), but all attempts were to no avail.

An hour later, after running out of ideas and because I had a deadline to meet, in desperation I asked Monet out-loud to please allow the printing to continue, since I had no intention of my work being published. As if by magic, the printer miraculously kicked into action, juddering into life again, completing the total task in hand. Mike and I looked at each other in disbelief but we were delighted at the intervention.

During the Christmas holidays, three years ago, our family came to stay, as is our usual tradition even though we were ill with a cold virus. It was during this time when I thought about my personal Tutor (from the time I was studying for my Degree), just wondering what he was doing since he was a very successful sculptor. I was shocked to read, when searching on the internet that he had died from leukaemia more than seven years earlier. I felt very sad at the loss of such a sensitive, talented artist who passed at the early age of fifty-seven.

Over that festive season, Richard 'tuned in' to me during my meditation time, when I understood he wanted me to contact his wife. He was very persistent. I had the impression she was depressed and in great need of contact and reassurance so I promised to write. On his fourth and last visit, I just saw Richard's face at my bedroom door. Due to my being ill and also lack of sleep, I told him to go away and that I would contact his wife when I felt able to do so.

When I had recovered, I wrote a long letter to his wife, Rebecca, talking about Richard's attributes as a Tutor and artist, also including photographs and amusing stories from our University group trip to Russia. I purposely avoided Richard's 'visitations' because Rebecca was a complete stranger to me and so I was not sure of her response to my letter.

It was about four days later, Rebecca wrote a lovely long letter to me, saying how she had laughed out loud when she had read my mail and she wanted us to meet up so she could give me a few keepsakes.

The next day, Rebecca wrote again to say Richard had woke her up that morning to give her lots of ideas on how to move forward in her life because she had been having 'a quiet time' (Rebecca's words), but Richard wanted her to 'get her boots on'.

Once I knew Rebecca was now in spiritual contact with Richard, I wrote back immediately to tell her about the four visitations I had had from Richard and about his insistence on making contact with her, such was his concern. He knew by contacting me, he could get his message through to her. Rebecca then told me when Richard was very ill, he said he would come back and haunt her, but Rebecca was afraid of this suggestion at the time.

I then wrote a more spiritual letter to Rebecca, about being a spiritual being having a human experience and that I believe Richard is still creating his work on another realm, just on a higher vibration. He now wants Rebecca to get involved with his work, collecting it from various museums, in order to organise a large exhibition.

The last time I heard from Rebecca, she was so very positive about life, having now, after ten years, removed her wedding ring and was about to embark on many new adventures. On reflection, I am sure this is what Richard wanted for Rebecca, to start to live again, rather than sinking into deep depression. I have not had any more contact with either Rebecca or Richard, so I realise all is well.

It is usually during the nightly meditating sessions when I have chats with various guides and relatives and it was on one such occasion my recently deceased brother came through for a short while. He told me he was still playing Jazz, as he used to love music in his earth time, but now he was pushing himself further by actually composing his own music. This was a bit of a surprise to hear since he had never talked about furthering his career in this direction, while he was living on this dimension. However, I was pleased to hear him say how happy he was in his new realm and then he faded away to allow someone else to 'come in'.

Last year, I awoke early due to having a slightly troubling dream about my brother, so I then meditated and was told I could talk to him if I wished. All I had to do was 'call him up' because if you wish to make contact with those family or friends over in the spirit world, just mention their name or look at their photo, while thinking about them, then they communicate with you instantly. After giving my brother a big hug, as he came through, we chatted for about thirty minutes when he was explaining about his current music, also that the scenery over there was stunning and the birdsong amazing. My brother always loved to cycle in the countryside when he was on our physical plane but now, he still often cycles, accompanying our Mum and Dad on their tandem, like when they were young. He commented our parents only look in their late twenties or early thirties now. (With this statement, I thought how wonderful that we are able to regain our youth and continue with our pleasurable activities, no longer being ill or infirm).

My brother continued to tell me he was now playing music with his long-standing friend, who had since passed over, (something I was not aware of) and another friend will not be too long passing. He went on to relate personal details of my future and then mentioned he was with us on our recent visit to Australia, when we were inspecting our son's new powerful sports car, (another of my brother's interests) and he was amused to see Mike and my other son having a test drive in the forest. Gordon was also impressed with the other new car belonging to our son who lives in the UK. My brother visits our grandson who attends a beautiful old boarding school in Dorset, when he mentioned how he loved the old buildings and commented how lucky our grandson was to secure a scholarship to such a school. He then went on to foretell a bit about the future career success of our grandson.

Towards the end of our conversation, my brother referred to his now deceased spouse, commenting she was well but he prefers not to be too close. He has forgiven her for what happened on the physical plane but his life is full and happy now, without stress. I was then given a farewell hug before he drifted off.

It felt so good afterwards, just as if my brother had popped in for a cup of tea, with his usual greeting, "Hello, 'ello, 'ello!", as he frequently did after one of his long cycling trips.

Chapter 2

Heightened Vibrations

and Consciousness

I agree with the author Omraam Mikael Aivanhov in his book 'Creation: Artistic and Spiritual' that a true artist is a priest, philosopher and scientist because the task of the artist is to interpret the world of spirit so it becomes embodied in substance on the physical world. However, this is easier said than done. It is exceedingly difficult to convey those 'feelings' into two dimensional and three-dimensional materials, hence the increased time meditating, in an effort to raise vibrations and consciousness. I believe painters, sculptors, musicians and poets have applied these methods in order to pass their knowledge within their masterpieces onto humanity, but only after the artist has completed a great deal of work on himself before commencing to create. This happens in a similar way when healing or performing Reiki. A few minutes prior to the healing are spent asking for assistance so you are able to channel the healing energy.

It is fascinating to realise that people are somehow drawn to looking at beauty, whether it is looking at artefacts in museums, exhibitions, galleries, libraries, or films etc. Almost subconsciously looking for the spiritual interpretation in the artefacts.

Patanjali, a sage in Hinduism, who is thought to be the author of a number of Sanskrit works more than 2,000 years ago, suggested, in order to define yourself:

"Dormant forces, faculties, and talents come alive, and you discover yourself to be a greater person by far than you ever dreamed yourself to be."

He was referring to the energy you feel when you are inspired. I can relate to this feeling of heightened excitement when I talk about my artwork. When I am on the right frequency, I feel so enthusiastic, so full of ideas and vibrancy. It just feels so right and as time and experiences increase along the way, I realise that I too am far stronger and more able than ever I thought, as the feeling of Spirit is working through me. This assistance is open to all, if only we learn how to access those forces.

Chapter 3

Lingering Energies in Buildings, Objects and Places

I find it fascinating to realise just how energies effect the whole interiors of buildings, the furniture, the fabrics and even the energies of people who used to live in the property. This experience of knowing if it is either a happy environment or a more negative place, is apparent as soon as I enter a home, no matter what the age of the building, both old and new alike.

From time to time, in my home, I am regularly aware of a certain floral fragrance and yet there are no flowers nearby. Firstly, it smelt like sweet tobacco, something both my husband and son have noticed too. I thought it may have been a visit from my Granddad, who passed over more than sixty years ago, because he used to smoke a pipe, using a similar fragrance of tobacco.

However, I have now noticed another different floral fragrance frequently, but this has not been noticed by other members of my family. I can only think this must be some message for me, maybe a guide wishing to communicate some information. I need to take heed. Oh, just as I am writing this sentence, there, I can smell the floral fragrance again. I know, at times during meditation, I have been aware of a sound like a choir of angels singing high up in the distance. It is not only my sense of smell but my hearing has become acute too, even more so as I am older. In fact, all my senses are now becoming more sensitive, hence the new experiences.

I have noticed that those people who have lost their sight, develop an acute sense of hearing and touch. It is as if they are no longer distracted from what is happening around them because they have lost the sense of sight.

About forty years ago, our house was up for sale as we were to move to a more rural location. There was great excitement as Mike and I arranged a viewing, but as soon as I entered the property, I became crest-fallen at the immense feeling of conflict, arguments, great rows and an overwhelming feeling of sadness. This home was full of negative energy, so needless to say, we did not buy the house. Our Estate Agent later informed us that the couple were in the throes of a divorce and so they needed to sell the house.

Other times, as members of the National Trust for many years, our family have regularly visited old buildings, and so quite often I have had to make a quick retreat if I happen to pick up on any negative energy. However, I also pick up on some wonderful energies too, with lovely warm feelings emanating around such places.

I remember one such incident when, years ago, I used to sell jumpers at 'House Parties', to raise a little pocket money when I was staying at home with my children. One of the parties was held in a dark, grey, deprived area and so I was not looking forward to the event. I need not have been concerned because as soon as I entered the house, I was met with a very heartfelt welcome. Once inside, the energy was so bright, vibrant and warm, I felt I was at the sea-side on a hot summer's day. Even forty years later, I have not forgotten the immense contrast of energy suspended in the most unlikely of places.

One summertime, our young family were on holiday down south, when we visited a very old cottage in the middle of the New Forest. I remember it was a sunny Saturday afternoon as we approached the red brick cottage, entering by the side of the house, through a turnstile, after buying our tickets. Our two young boys were very playful at the time, scampering around the lovely garden, before we entered the cottage on a guided tour.

The property was quite small, full of visitors as we climbed the rickety stairs, only to find beds of straw and where about twelve children used to live with their parents. The tour continued downstairs, into the kitchen as the interesting chat continued. Then we followed into a small sitting room with a black fireplace. As soon as I entered this room, I became enveloped with a feeling of horror, a frightening energy. I just had to get out of there as quick as I could, only to find, when out in the sunny garden, I was unable to answer Mike's questions as to what was the matter. I was unable to speak, because I was in so much shock. It took about twenty minutes before my voice returned, when I was able to relay the shocking details of what had happened in that room. Although I had previously had reactions to negative energy, I had never before, or since, lost my voice. Mike wanted us to leave the premises immediately, but I thought this was ridiculous, on such a bright sunny day, not even thinking about such violence. So, I decided to go into the property alone this time, just to see what happened. As soon as I went into the sitting-room, I became consumed with fear. I knew a child had died in that room. I felt she had been thrown onto the fire, in rage and she had died as a result of this violent attack. Once outside, I composed myself then decided to find someone who could explain the negative energy. Since it was lunchtime, there were no guides available, but I managed to find the ticket collector who was at the turnstile. I tentatively asked if anything had actually happened in the past to a family member in that small sitting room. I was told a young child died in there after accidently falling on the fire. It is my own opinion that I believe the incident was far more traumatic and that it was not an accident. I think the child was actually pushed onto the fire.

To celebrate my sixtieth Birthday, Mike and I visited Prague for a short holiday. We stayed in a beautiful hotel, housed in a very old building, with a spacious luxurious dining room where we ate our meal to the sound of beautiful music being played on a Baby Grand piano. The stage was set for a wonderful Birthday treat.

However, as we later strolled around the city, I began to feel very uneasy. The atmosphere felt very dark and sinister, an emotion I had experienced in other negative spaces. As we walked on the bridge, crossing the river, I bought some very stylish jewellery from a small stall, earrings and matching necklace, made from the local green slate. Although I was drawn to the decorative pieces, they never felt good to hold, because of the negative energy emitting from them, so on my return home, I gave them away.

I was so relieved to leave this place and yet, on my arrival home, my daughter informed me that some of the cobblestones in the street were actually made up of the gravestones of the Jewish people who used to live there and their names and details were hidden on the underside of the cobbles. Mike has since told me that during World War 11, the Jewish people were marched over the bridge to their deaths in mass graves, where I had bought the jewellery. I had not known those facts but it is no wonder I was picking up so much negative energy.

Last year, Mike and I were touring Yorkshire and so on our way home, we decided to stay overnight at a very old Coaching Inn in Harrogate.

Our meal in the restaurant was delicious and yet, as soon as we were shown to our room, I felt as if I had walked into a wall of negativity. My whole body started to vibrate and I could not settle, so I requested another room. The landlady kindly led me into the only other two available rooms and yet I had the same violent response. This was such a different energy to the benevolent one in the restaurant downstairs, where my body began to settle down again. Even though it was late in the evening, by this time, I realised I was unable to stay in any of those rooms, with such sinister energy. I was so desperate, I even considered sleeping in our car but Mike insisted we return home that night, arriving in the early hours. I remember it took about an hour for my body to stop vibrating due to that very menacing atmosphere.

Just on leaving the Coaching Inn, I went to the bar in order to return our room key. Immediately I saw the landlord, an image of a Highwayman overlaid his persona. This was the first time I had experienced this instant impression of someone's past life. Even now, after all this time, I still have no doubts of this man's earlier life and this may explain why he was so happy and comfortable in that old Inn.

Now I realise my sensitivity to certain environments is forever increasing, I need to be more vigilant when entering certain properties. I know I pick up on negative energies if there has been lots of physical and verbal abuse in a household and I still vividly remember the terror I felt when entering that old cottage in the New Forest almost forty years earlier.

It was about thirty-five years ago, our family were invited to a huge family celebration in Godmanchester, in Cambridgeshire for the occasion of Mike's Uncle's seventieth Birthday. The family is extremely large and so members in our local community were transported by coach to join in the festivities.

With the party in full swing, in this beautiful Georgian house and gardens, Mike's cousin invited me to look around the old property, much of it having been lovingly restored by Julia. We both have much in common, having a love of making soft furnishings and so I was extremely interested to see the fruits of her labour, the newly reconditioned window seat, the beautifully restored fireplace, having been found hidden behind a dreadful modern one, etc.

As we chatted away, I was now standing in the doorway of Julia's bedroom, when I came over feeling extremely cold, as if there was an icy draught from an open window and yet it was a wonderful warm, sunny afternoon. Julia took one look at my face and asked what was the matter because my whole expression had changed. As I explained about the sudden icy chill, she then told me I was standing in exactly the same place where she often sees a spirit lady from the past, dressed in white.

One summer, Mike and I decided to tour Scotland. I remember one sunny Saturday during this holiday, we stopped at Fort William to have a look around at what seemed like a busy market. It took a while to find a space on the car park, but as soon as I got out of the car, I suddenly felt very unwell. This feeling was instant and one I recognised as negative energy. Due to this great discomfort, I decided I needed to leave this place immediately, even though we had only just arrived. This was much to Mike's frustration, but he understood my sensitivity to such atmospheres.

Once we had travelled some distance away, Mike then told me a little of the history of Fort William, that there had been a great massacre between the Redcoats and the Scottish soldiers around 1746. This was something I had not been aware of because I had not studied History at school. I had instantly picked up on the horror and negative energy emanating in the area of Fort William, even though the battles were more than two hundred and seventy years earlier.

Another day on this same holiday, Mike and I decided to go on a hike within the forest. The weather was fine when we set off, but usual to Scotland, the rain started as drizzle and progressed to a downpour. However, we were well prepared for every eventuality, wearing good waterproofs, hiking boots and carrying rucksacks.

Our walk started to lead us up a steep hill within the forest, when I became aware of the cobble stones underfoot. I continued to climb on this slippery path, in the pouring rain, when I noticed a strong smell of tobacco smoke. This was most intriguing since there were no other people around, only us two, who are non-smokers. It was then that Mike, who is extremely knowledgeable about history, explained we were actually walking on an old military road, used by the soldiers and horses to pull along the cannon. I believe the lingering smell of tobacco was still around from the soldiers, who may have been stopping for a rest and a smoke, while labouring with the military hardware.

Those accounts above are just a few examples of how our energies remain in our environment, even though many years have passed.

Chapter 4

Symbols From the Spirit World

Throughout history it is interesting to observe how us humans often turn to nature to reflect on symbolic incidents in our lives. For example, I was walking deep in the forest one cool wintery February day, when I noticed a red admiral butterfly began to join us on our walk. It fluttered along with us, for several hundred metres, waiting for us to catch up with it, while resting on the bushes along the pathway. I was taken aback because I had never seen butterflies out in such cold weather. It was then I began to realise it may have been my brother, who had very recently passed away. He too loved country walks and so may have joined us. On our way back through the forest, as we headed home, the red admiral re-joined us once again, almost to say 'farewell'.

Recently, my husband had been given a tank experience as a gift from the family. While we were awaiting his turn, as there were six tanks in operation during that afternoon, we sauntered around the tanks and military paraphernalia which were exhibited in a enclosed museum. As we were in a windowless room, full of uniforms, guns, helmets, ammunition and the like, I commented that my brother would have liked to be in here too, since for years he had collected artefacts from both World War 1 and World War

11, having visited the battlefields of the Somme and other areas. He often shared army stories with my husband, and viewed films together since my Mike used to be in the army and so they had a common interest.

Suddenly, we were aware of a black butterfly constantly fluttering around us, up and down the room for several minutes. There were no other people in the room, or even any windows. We both then remembered our winter walk in the forest, when a butterfly had accompanied us, believing it to represent my brother who had recently passed over. Once again, my husband and I thought my brother had again joined us in the tank museum.

Mike thoroughly enjoyed his hour-long tank session, trundling around a huge field with the six other vehicles, creating huge dust clouds, almost like a desert scene. As he walked towards me, my husband looked rather pensive when he said, "You're not going to believe what I am about to tell you, but a butterfly flew alongside my tank for the whole hour, six circuits around the field!". We believe this may have been my brother, enjoying the trip with Mike. In fact, we have looked closely at the photographs to try to see the insect, but unfortunately, we were not able to see it due to the great clouds of dust created by the tanks.

Later, we went to a local pub for lunch, when indoors, a very large cricket hopped onto my shoulder after our meal. My husband gently removed him and took the insect outside. I have since read that crickets are a symbol of good luck.

Two weeks later, we met friends for a day walking in the Derbyshire Dales, where later in the afternoon, we had tea in the sunny cafe garden. As we chatted, I became aware of a butterfly circling our table several times, before settling down on my coffee cup. (The cup was still full of hot coffee). Is someone trying to tell me something? Is my brother still around? He would have loved to cycle in those rugged Dales, something he would do on a regular basis, and also stop off for a refreshing cup of tea in that sunny garden.

Chapter 5

Meeting other Psychics

A few years ago, I was visiting a Wellbeing Show in Birmingham, when on impulse, I made an appointment to chat with one of the mediums present at the show. There was a list of about thirty of them, from which to choose and as I quickly glanced around the area, I made my choice. Little did I know at the time, that Annie was also an artist and so we had so much in common, it seemed as if we were not strangers. I was told I needed to get my work out in the public arena and to contact certain Societies to obtain suitable spaces. Annie accurately described my home, with its spiritual shelf, where I display my family photos of those in spirit, a plant, candle and a Buddha figure too. By this time, I was very impressed with her precision and even more so now, because her prediction of how I will have to be very careful on what food I eat, has certainly come to fruition.

As I was finishing my day at this exhibition, at one of the last stands, a young woman approached me and insisted I take one of the ribbons from her basket. I was tired by this time and refused her offer, but she held my hand and drew me in closer saying she needed to talk to me. She said I needed to take one step at a time towards enlightenment. I was rather taken aback because those were exactly the same words used by Annie, although I stayed silent to see what would ensue with this meeting. I was told I was very psychic and that I need to use this gift. My Grandma then appeared, in spirit, and pinned some white Lily of the Valley flowers to my left side, with silver paper underneath and then attached some Lavender too.

This medium, Alison, commented how much I looked like my Grandma, something my Mum had always said and that we would get on like a 'house on fire'. The medium continued to say that Grandma is often at our home, (I know), and that my recently deceased brother was now by her side. Well, I was shocked and a little upset by this comment because I had not mentioned it earlier about my sibling passing away, so I then began to open up, offering a little information. I said there had been no funeral for my brother, who lived abroad, and I was not told about his pending death, his ashes were sent out to sea and his personal effects were stolen. It was a dreadful story. Alison then said my brother kept repeating one word, "Spiteful, spiteful".

I then explained that my brothers' wife had now passed too, but Alison said she is not with my brother because he is with our Mum, Dad and Grandma. This statement corresponds with my meditative sessions with my brother and I was so impressed with Alison's accuracy, I made a mental note to visit her at her home at a later date.

In the meantime, I looked up the significance of the flowers I had kindly received from my Grandma. The Lily of the Valley is a symbol of gently wakening us through harmonising our nervous system, including the brain, with the multidimensional frequencies. While Lavender works through the energy circuits in the brain that interpret incoming information. The combination of the two flowers result in a calm mind, so it is impossible to be unnerved by anything.

It was about a month later when I met up with Alison again. She too, like Annie, said it was important to get my work out in the public arena. In the past, I had been gently held back, but now it was my time and so I need to set a time each day to produce my work because I have much to do. I was also advised to include Mike in set tasks of assisting with the logistics, exhibiting etc. He has always been supportive throughout my journey, as I knew it was important to include him in my endeavours, otherwise, we would be living entirely different lives and not spending time together.

Alison then confirmed that Mike and I had lived many lives together, which we had suspected, since we were only young children when we met this time around. Even then, Mike said he knew instantly that we would be together in this life. The medium then talked about our family, confirming that one of my grandsons is a 'star child,' being from Lemuria, the sunken continent of an ancient civilization. I have always known him to be gifted and special, even with his understanding of healing and psychic happenings when he was only four years old.

I then mentioned that the previous day, Mike and I were working on a healing session, when he commented that Mary Ann is here. Being born in the Victorian era, my Grandma sternly corrected him with, "It's Mrs. Mills to you". Alison then added, "She didn't like him showing her his bits either!!" Wow! This was actually true but I had omitted to tell Alison the whole conversation from Mary-Ann. It was my Grandma in spirit who had told her. The previous morning, after a shower, Mike commenced his healing session, but he was draped in a bath towel and yet Grandma came through sternly to remind him to wear clothes next time. Mike and I giggled about this at the time and yet Mike has always heeded her advice ever since, whenever he's healing. This was such a private moment, I never realised that Grandma would share this information with another stranger, although she being a medium. Beware!

As our session was drawing to a close, Alison asked Mike about the two feathers he wore down behind his left ear, white feathers, tipped with black, as he used to belong to the Dakota Sioux tribe. Alison was talking about one of Mike's past lives. He was so surprised with this description, because this confirmed the information he received from White Eagle, during his time in America.

Chapter 6

Spirit Activity at Home and Away

Last month, Mike decided to have an early night and go to bed, while I sat watching the television. As he was cleaning his teeth in the bathroom, with the door wide open, he saw my spirit Grandma climbing our stairs, then walk across the landing and walk into our bedroom. She appeared as a young woman, dressed in Victorian clothing i.e. a white frilly, long sleeved blouse, with frills around the neck and a smart long navy skirt. Mike was so taken aback with this striking figure, he followed my Grandma into our room, with his toothbrush still in his hand. However, my Grandma was nowhere to be seen.

This is not the first time my Grandma has appeared to Mike and yet I am not surprised to know she is around, because I have often felt a presence and a Psychic also said she visits us often. It was three years ago, when Mike was washing up in our kitchen, he thought he saw me, wearing my long blue dressing gown, passing the door in our hall. He started to chat to me but there was no response. He then looked in the hall to see where I had gone, only to find I was actually having a shower in the bathroom. Only then did he begin to realise he must have seen Grandma, visiting us, while wearing her long blue dress.

While our children were young, we went to Bournemouth each year, staying at the same Guest House, then hiring a beach hut so the children were able to play on the sand each day. Our family used to look forward to this annual treat.

One time, for our accommodation, we were given the room over the dining room, in this old Victorian house, when, during the night, I was suddenly awoken by a dreadful, sinister feeling of a man, dressed in black, wearing a tall top hat, leaning closely over the bed, towards me. This felt a very threatening, negative energy. So much so, my heart was beating so very fast and although I had woken Mike, it still took me a long time to eventually fall asleep, making a mental note, not to stay in that same room again on our next visit.

At breakfast, I asked the owner if there had been any 'spiritual happenings' within the house, something she denied, but then I understood, because an admission would have been detrimental for business.

The following year, I made yet another reservation at this same Guest House with the request for a different room from the previous year, one at the top of the property. By this time, the Guest House had been sold and the new owner, David, was very pleasant but new to the hospitality business. That summer, we made friends with a middle-aged couple, Pat and Dan, who were staying in the same accommodation, in the room over the dining room, where the previous year, I had experienced that frightening episode. Obviously, I did not mention this to our newly acquainted friends.

Later that week, following a day on the beach together with our new friends, our family entered the dining room at a pre-arranged time and Pat then joined us. Dan was following shortly. As the diners were sitting quietly, there was an almighty crash from above the dining room. The whole house shuddered and the diners, being shocked into silence, looked upwards to the ceiling.

After a while, Dan appeared, his face ashen, still in shock, while the guests eagerly awaited an explanation. It appears that Dan was sat on the bed, bending over to tie his shoelace, when the large heavy Jacobean wardrobe fell over towards him, crashing just short of Dan's head. He was very shocked because no one had touched or even used the wardrobe and so he could not understand why such a heavy piece of furniture could have fallen over. However, Dan realised he was very lucky to have escaped serious injury but I decided that this was not the time to mention my experience in that very same room, the previous year.

Later, when I was able to have a quiet chat with the new owner, David, out of the earshot of his other guests, he was far more relaxed and open about the odd happenings, rather than the previous owners of the business, which he and his family had been experiencing within the house. One time, he was awoken during the night to the sound of footsteps walking up and down in the room above his bedroom.   David feared there were intruders in the property, so he went upstairs, with his son, to investigate.

However, they were unable to find anyone. There were times when cutlery and water jugs had disappeared and so David replaced them only after a thorough search of the house and dustbins. There was no evidence of broken glass from the jugs or missing cutlery. Also, one night, David was decorating the room where Dan and I had experienced those unusual happenings and he had left a pot of paint suspended on top of the ladders. After a while, the pot of paint started swinging at a great pace. Dan was very open about discussing such incidents in the Guest House and so I shared my experiences too.

Spirit Activity at Home.

Since our family live great distances from us, it is only about every three months when we make an effort to travel to meet up together. (Our daughter lives in Hampshire, a son in Surrey, while our eldest son lives with his family in Australia). On one such occasion, following lunch, those of us in the UK, gathered around to watch a particular television programme. The silence was broken by the sudden clattering of a family Wedding photo, as it fell off the wall onto the radiator. This was the photo of our son's wedding i.e. the one who lives in Australia. This picture had been on our wall for twenty-five years, only being moved when we were decorating the room. It was as if our son in Australia was connecting with the comment, 'now we are **all** together'.

A few weeks ago, I was packing clothes ready to visit our family down south, just for a few days. As I was sorting out my fashion necklaces, I was looking for one of my favourites, not expensive, but a North American Indian artefact, made from a wooden seed pod, cut cross section with an image of a howling wolf, cut out by a laser.

I slowly trawled through my necklaces three times, which were hanging on several hooks on my wardrobe door, but I was still unable to find my treasured possession. I then searched through my bedside cabinet and another bedroom, all to no avail. Since I was rather upset, Mike then also carefully looked through the large number of trinkets a couple of times, but he too could not find my special one.

Later, I sat on the bed and asked St. Anthony to help me find it. I heard a voice saying, 'Go back again and look in the wardrobe'. As I followed the instruction, I slowly opened the door and there, on top of my necklaces, on the very first hook, in full view was my wolf necklace!! I was shocked and delighted. Thank you again, St Anthony.

www.ingramcontent.com/pod-product-compliance
Lightning Source LLC
Chambersburg PA
CBHW071124220526
45467CB00004B/2053

* 9 7 9 8 3 9 0 3 6 0 1 3 2 *